HISTAMINE INTOLERANCE
FOOD LIST

Take this book everywhere!

D1715628

BY THE HISTAMINE HEROES

LEGAL & DISCLAIMER

HOW TO USE THIS FOOD LIST

This book works like a dictionary. Look for a food, drink or ingredient alphabetically or on search.

Once you find what you are looking for, it is scored between 1 and 5 for histamine levels based on careful analysis of the world's best sources (listed below) for histamine intolerance.

- 5 indicates the least amount of histamine (or histamine-releasing or DAO blocking)

- 1 indicates the most amount of histamine (or histamine-releasing or DAO blocking)

So on a low-histamine diet, 5 is best and 1 is worst. You would look to be initially consuming more 5 foods and cutting out 1 foods. As time goes on, with the help of a skilled practitioner, you would look to be reintroducing as many foods as possible to get a varied and nutritious diet.

We decided on a scoring system between 1 and 5 as many food lists only group foods into 'high' or 'low' histamine, and we felt there was considerably more nuance to histamine in food and drink than this. The most respected sites often disagree on major foods and this is unsurprising as histamine varies so often portion to portion and person to person, so we've tried to reflect that in our list.

As Yasmina Ykelenstam noted on the site 'Healing Histamine', for every food eliminated, one "safe" food should be added into the diet. Otherwise, you could soon be heading down the scary path of orthorexia – a type of anorexia based on the demonization of certain foods.

We whole-heartedly agree with these sentiments. Our aim is to heal from histamine intolerance, and live a healthy, balanced life in every aspect. Keep this book close by when you cook or eat out, and dip in and out whenever you need to check if something is low histamine.

SOURCES

These excellent sources are very highly recommended in your further research on histamine intolerance. As far as possible we have consulted all these sites in our research into this food list. They vary considerably which is the reason why we wrote this book. This entire book comes with the caveat that absolutely everybody reacts differently to certain foods, and therefore histamine food lists are difficult to compile (and quite important as a result). Please do click on the below sites for further reading.

- Histamine Intolerance Awareness Site Food List - https://www.histamineintolerance.org.uk/about/the-food-diary/the-food-list/

- Alison Vickery Anti-Food List - https://www.alisonvickery.com/blog/anti-histamine-foods

- SFGATE Histamine Reducing Foods - https://healthyeating.sfgate.com/histaminereducing-foods-12197.html

- Factvsfitness Master List Of Low Histamine Foods - https://factvsfitness.com/blogs/news/histamine-intolerance-food-list

- SIGHI Food List - https://www.mastzellaktivierung.info/downloads/foodlist/21_FoodList_EN_alphabetic_withCateg.pdf

- The Histamine Intolerance Site Food List (referenced throughout with permission) https://histamineintolerance.net/foodlist

- MastCell360 Low and High Histamine Food Lists https://mastcell360.com/low-histamine-foods-list/

- Healing Histamine, Histamine In Food Lists https://healinghistamine.com/what-is-histamine/histamine-in-food-lists/

BRIEF INTRODUCTION

Congratulations on choosing this book. We wrote it because we suffer from histamine intolerance ourselves, and we were frustrated at how so much information out there seems to confuse us and conflict with other sources. So we decided to take the world's best and most trusted histamine intolerance lists and guides and compile the information into one easy-to-consult guide.

We know that this list is not perfect, because that's the nature of histamine intolerance. Everybody reacts differently, and foods even show up differently depending on the growing process, their freshness or ripeness, and of course, how long they've been sitting in the fridge for. But we believe it is the most comprehensive out there.

We're not going to chew over the reasons behind your histamine intolerance. You've almost certainly done your research on it, and that's why you are here in the first place, for the most comprehensive food list available on histamine intolerance.

Suffice to say that histamine is implicated in every allergy response process, including food allergies. They work to cause a reaction when you consume something you react to. Most people don't have to worry about this, but a sizeable minority (up to 15% of us) do. And that's why it's worth having a really detailed histamine intolerance food list.

If you have allergies, no matter what kind, use this book to avoid foods that are high in histamine, histamine-releasing, or inhibit the production of DAO. These include alcohol, leftovers, aged foods, preservatives, fermented foods and more. You'll learn all about what to avoid from this book, and you might start to feel a lot better from your histamine intolerance.

We hope to have made a meaningful contribution with this book.

Please keep in mind that materials and resources like this book are no substitute for medical advice and not intended as such.

Still, we are convinced it will make your life a little easier.

THE FOOD LIST

Acerola: 4

- Histamine Intolerance Site: ✅ (Green - low histamine)
- Comments: Cherries tend to be lower histamine but there is sometimes some debate. See other comments on 'Cherry'. Could be high in oxalates.

Agave Syrup: 5

- Histamine Intolerance Site: ✅ (Green - low histamine)
- Comments: Consume in moderation. A lower sugar diet is generally healthier. This also applies to agave nectar.

Alcohol: 1

- Histamine Intolerance Site: 😠 (Red - high histamine)
- Comments: Alcohols are some of the most problematic things you can consume on a low histamine diet. The Healing Histamine Site notes that alcohol itself isn't always high histamine but has the effect of blocking DAO (diamine oxidase) production. The prospect of giving up alcohol often comes as a bit of a shock to people starting a histamine diet for the first time. Don't be disheartened if you are new to this. Start by cutting out alcohol and once you reduce your histamine levels re-introduce slowly. Wines are often extremely problematic although some low-histamine wines can be found. But note the DAO-

blocking element above. Alcohols contain histaminic-degrading enzymes, but some rums, tequilas and Tito's Vodka may be purer than others. We have seen some claims online that plain vodka, gin and white rum are all low in histamine - these may be better options than other alcohols, but they still may block your DAO enzyme and therefore cause a histamine reaction.

Algae: 1

- Histamine Intolerance Site: 😠 (Red - high histamine)
- Comments: A number of supplements contain algae and we have found these to cause a reaction too.

Almond: 3

- Histamine Intolerance Site: 😕 (yellow - medium histamine)

- Comments: According to Mast Cell 360, small amounts are well tolerated. This is one of those foods that we have found we tolerate well at times. At others, it causes a reaction. As always with histamine intolerance, everybody is different. With almonds test in very small quantities initially.

Anchovies: 1

- Histamine Intolerance Site: 😠 (Red - high histamine)
- Comments: Most fish are very high histamine. Ideally fish should be frozen within one hour of catching, and even

then anchovies are poorly tolerated. Other fish may be better.

Anise: 2

- Histamine Intolerance Site: 😕 (yellow - medium histamine)

- Comments:

Apple: 1

- Histamine Intolerance Site: ✅ (green - low histamine)

- Comments: Apples are thought to potentially lower your histamine levels.

Apple Cider Vinegar: 3

- Histamine Intolerance Site: 😕 (yellow - medium histamine)

- Comments: The best tolerated vinegar. Many find this acceptable. If it doesn't suit you, search for something called 'verjus' which may work in a similar way.

Apricot: 5

- Histamine Intolerance Site: ✅ (green - low histamine)

- Comments: Who doesn't love apricot? Eat in moderation as higher in sugar.

Artichoke: 5

- Histamine Intolerance Site: ✅ (green - low histamine)
- Comments:

Artificial Sweeteners: 1

- Histamine Intolerance Site: 😠 (red - high histamine)
- Comments: There are so many health reasons why you want to be avoiding artificial sweeteners. There is much we don't know about their effects on the body. Stick to natural sweeteners like stevia.

Asparagus: 5

- Histamine Intolerance Site: ✅ (green - low histamine)
- Comments: Lots of veggies are great on a low-histamine diet, and asparagus is one of those.

Aubergine (Eggplant): 2

- Histamine Intolerance Site: 😠 (red - high histamine)
- Comments: Wait, did we just say lots of veggies are good? Yes, but not all veggies are created equal. Unfortunately aubergine comes up high on the major food lists. Fruits and vegetables with peels tend to be high in histamines.

Avocado: 1

- Histamine Intolerance Site: 😠 (red - high histamine)

- Comments: This is one of the major disappointment for people starting out on a low histamine diet for the first time. It almost seems incomprehensible that avocados could not be healthy. But often they are very high in histamine levels particularly ones that are very soft. Avoid or treat with extreme caution. This includes avocado oil although apparently it is lower in histamine if cold pressed.

Bamboo Shoots: 3

- Histamine Intolerance Site: 😕 (yellow - medium histamine)
- Comments:

Banana: 2

- Histamine Intolerance Site: 😠 (red - high histamine)
- Comments: Bananas can often be very high in histamine. It's thought that the younger/greener, the better you will tolerate it, so avoid ripe bananas.

Barbary Fig: 3

- Histamine Intolerance Site: 😕 (yellow - medium histamine)
- Comments:

Barley: 3

- Histamine Intolerance Site: 😕 (yellow – medium histamine)

- Comments: Barley seems to be tolerated generally quite well. However it contains gluten and many people who are low histamine will follow a gluten-free diet and therefore will want to avoid Barley

Barley Malt, Malt: 2

- Histamine Intolerance Site: 😠 (red - high histamine)
- Comments: Different from barley as fermented, which is a big no-no in histamine.

Basil: 5

- Histamine Intolerance Site: ✅ (green - low histamine)
- Comments: Delicious. We love making a basil pesto with olive oil and small amount of almonds.

Bay laurel, laurel: 3

- Histamine Intolerance Site: 😕 (yellow - medium histamine)
- Comments:

Beans: 1

- Histamine Intolerance Site: 😠 (red - high histamine)
- Comments: Ugh, beans and histamine intolerance don't often go together. Everybody is different and there may be exceptions but we generally don't react well to them.

Beef: 5

- Histamine Intolerance Site: ✅ (green - low histamine)
- Comments: There are a few rules here. It should be organic - in fact must be, so that you avoid fertilisers and pesticides. It's also – and this is the big issue – must not be aged. Next time you are in a steak restaurant to take a close look at the menu. You'll see that most of the cuts of meat on there are actually aged and therefore will be high and histamine. However if you can find some fresh beef that is organic then you are good to go.

Beer: 1

- Histamine Intolerance Site: 😠 (red - high histamine)
- Comments: See our comments on alcohol.

Beetroot: 5

- Histamine Intolerance Site: ✅ (green - low histamine)
- Comments:

Bell Pepper (Hot): 2

- Histamine Intolerance Site: 😠 (red - high histamine)
- Comments: Some may be okay with bell peppers. Test very carefully.

Bell Pepper (Sweet): 1

- Histamine Intolerance Site: ✅ (green - low histamine)

- Comments: High in pesticide residue according to Mast Cell 360, buy organic. (This applies really to all foods - but especially foods which collect more pesticide. We tend to buy all our produce organic, which means we'll never be rich, but we will be healthier!)

Bison: 5

- Histamine Intolerance Site: ✅ (green - low histamine)
- Comments: Must not be aged. Same as beef, high in histamines if aged. We would love to eat more bison but struggle to source it where we live. It's a good alternative to beef with less saturated fat.

Bivalves (Mussels, Oyster, Clams, Scallops): 1

- Histamine Intolerance Site: 😠 (red – high histamine)
- Comments: Bad news for seafood lovers. (Who knew these seafoods were called bivalves?)

Black Caraway: 5

- Histamine Intolerance Site: ✅ (green - low histamine)
- Comments: One of the good guys... its thought can help lower histamine levels.

Blackberry: 5

- Histamine Intolerance Site: ✅ (green - low histamine)
- Comments:

Blackcurrants: 5

- Histamine Intolerance Site: ✅ (green - low histamine)
- Comments:

Blue Cheeses: 1

- Histamine Intolerance Site: 😠 (red - high histamine)
- Comments: These blue cheeses are blue because they are mouldy and therefore high in histamine. There are other cheese options which are lower histamine and you can find them throughout this book. Take a look at ricotta cheese, cream cheese and soft cheese. You might also get on well with mozzarella.

Blue Fenugreek: 2

- Histamine Intolerance Site: 😠 (red - high histamine)
- Comments:

Blueberries: 5

- Histamine Intolerance Site: ✅ (green - low histamine)
- Comments: Some say blueberries are histamine fighting, which is good news.

Bok choi: 5

- Histamine Intolerance Site: ✅ (green - low histamine)

- Comments: Sometimes also written as *bok choy*. A lovely leafy green veg. Try sautéing or lightly roasting for 15 minutes.

Borlotti Beans: 2

- Histamine Intolerance Site: 😠 (red - high histamine)

- Comments: See our more general comments under *Beans*

Bouillon: 1

- Histamine Intolerance Site: 😠 (red – high histamine)

- Comments: Stocks are often high histamine if they're a bone broth of sorts. In addition, shop-bought ones can be a lot worse. According to SIGHI, its ingredients are almost always incompatible (glutamate, yeast extract, spice/ aroma/ flavor/ seasoning/ condiment, meat extracts, incompatible vegetables)

Boysenberry: 3

- Histamine Intolerance Site: 😕 (yellow - medium histamine)

- Comments:

Brandy: 1

- Histamine Intolerance Site: 😠 (red – high histamine)

- Comments: See "Alcohol"

Brazil Nut: 4

- Histamine Intolerance Site: ☑ (green - low histamine)
- Comments: Certain nuts can be high in histamine if moldy, but brazil nuts should be okay.

Bread: 3

- Histamine Intolerance Site: 😐 (yellow - medium histamine)
- Comments: listed as a '3' as we don't know the ingredients of each individual bread. Check the individual ingredients on our list in this book. Also fermentation process and yeasting process is uncertain but you may well tolerate most breads. Test with caution. You could even make your own!

Broad-Leaved Garlic: 4

- Histamine Intolerance Site: 😐 (yellow - medium histamine)
- Comments:

Broad Beans: 1

- Histamine Intolerance Site: 😠 (red – high histamine)
- Comments: See comments on 'Beans'. Also known as Vicia Faba.

Broccoli: 5

- Histamine Intolerance Site: ☑ (green - low histamine)

- Comments: So good for you. Enjoy.

Brussels Sprouts: 3

- Histamine Intolerance Site: 😕 (yellow – medium histamine)

- Comments: Some say Brussels sprouts are low histamine so it's very much worth testing them out. We like to buy them and freeze them and cook from frozen in the oven.

Buckwheat: 2

- Histamine Intolerance Site: 😡 (red - high histamine)

Butter: 5

- Histamine Intolerance Site: ✅ (green - low histamine)

- Comments: Organic, grass-fed butter is important. It's easy to find. Lots of the butter is in your local supermarket will hopefully be grass-fed, organic and affordable. Cultured butter is usually well-tolerated according to SIGHI.

Cabbage: 5

- Histamine Intolerance Site: ✅ (green - low histamine)

- Comments: We love cabbage. It's very versatile and (important one) very cheap, even organic. However, caution. Pickled cabbage is not good - the pickling makes it high-histamine.

Cactus Pear: 3

- Histamine Intolerance Site: 😕 (yellow – medium histamine)
- Comments:

Cardamom: 5

- Histamine Intolerance Site: ✅ (green - low histamine)
- Comments: Love cardamom so much. One of the most exotic spices. A nice way to add a little sweetness to recipes.

Carrot: 5

- Histamine Intolerance Site: ✅ (green - low histamine)
- Comments: More veggies on the 'good list'.

Cashew nut: 2

- Histamine Intolerance Site: 😕 (yellow - medium histamine)
- Comments: Experts vary on cashew nuts. Some lists suggest that they can be okay in small quantities. But we have listed it as a 2 out of 5 as we react and know other people who do too.

Cassava: 5

- Histamine Intolerance Site: ✅ (green - low histamine)

- Comments: Delicious as a flour and great gluten-free alternative.

Cauliflower: 5

- Histamine Intolerance Site: ✓ (green - low histamine)
- Comments:

Celery: 5

- Histamine Intolerance Site: ✓ (green - low histamine)
- Comments: Some say this can be histamine-lowering.

Cep Mushrooms: 2

- Histamine Intolerance Site: 😠 (red - high histamine)
- Comments: 'Shrooms massively vary from person to person and from mushroom to mushroom. Test carefully.

Chamomile And Chamomile Tea: 5

- Histamine Intolerance Site: ✓ (green - low histamine)
- Comments:

Champagne: 1

- Histamine Intolerance Site: 😠 (red - high histamine)
- Comments: see comments on 'Alcohol'.

Chard: 3

- Histamine Intolerance Site: 😕 (yellow - medium histamine)

- Comments: Swiss chard listed as low histamine. Oxalate issues please check with chard.

Cheddar Cheese: 1

- Histamine Intolerance Site: 😠 (red – high histamine)

- Comments: See comments on cheeses. Look for softer cheese alternatives.

Cheese Made From Unpasteurized "Raw" Milk: 1

- Histamine Intolerance Site: 😠 (red - high histamine)

- Comments: See comments on cheeses. Look for softer cheese alternatives.

Soft cheeses: 3

- Histamine Intolerance Site: 😕 (yellow – medium histamine)

- Comments: Soft cheeses tend to be much lower histamine options than hard cheeses and blue cheeses. The younger the cheese the less likely it is to be high and histamine or histamine releasing. Again as with everything involving histamine test extremely carefully. One batch of cheese will not be the same as another when it comes to histamine. Soft cheeses such as mozzarella ricotta and spreadable soft cheese may be tolerated.

Cheese: Hard Cheese, All Well Matured Cheeses: 1

- Histamine Intolerance Site: 😠 (red - high histamine)
- Comments: cheesy hell for histamine intolerance sufferers! Sad times for those of us who love cheese.

Cherry: 4

- Histamine Intolerance Site: ✅ (green - low histamine)
- Comments: Sometimes a debate about cherries. We buy ours frozen to lock in the nutrients and prevent any increase in histamine.

Chestnut: 5

- Histamine Intolerance Site: ✅ (green - low histamine)
- Comments: Includes sweet chestnut

Chia, Chia Seeds: 5

- Histamine Intolerance Site: ✅ (green - low histamine)
- Comments: Those with histamine stomach issues may want to soak a small amount of chia seeds first and eat in moderation.

Chicken: 5

- Histamine Intolerance Site: ✅ (green - low histamine)
- Comments: Must be organic and fresh, not leftovers. Generally, the longer food has been left to sit, the more histamine it has. Canned food, which takes many years to

expire, is the worst as far as histamine content is concerned. In summary canned chicken is terrible, organic freshly cooked chicken is great!

Chickpeas: 2

- Histamine Intolerance Site: 😠 (red - high histamine)
- Comments: We react particularly badly to chickpeas, and while that's just a personal opinion, the general vibe seems to be - avoid them.

Chicory: 5

- Histamine Intolerance Site: ✅ (green - low histamine)
- Comments:

Chili Pepper, Red, Fresh: 2

- Histamine Intolerance Site: 😠 (red - high histamine)
- Comments: Spicy foods can release histamine, which becomes an issue when added to the histamine produced by seasonal allergies or histamine intolerance. You could try to avoid spicy food when your histamine symptoms are acting up.

Chives: 4

- Histamine Intolerance Site: 😕 (yellow - medium histamine)
- Comments:

Chocolate: 2

- Histamine Intolerance Site: 😠 (red - high histamine)

- Comments: Chocolate is generally thought of being a histamine liberator rather than being high in histamine. This is clearly not good news. White chocolate can be tolerated a little better, but frustratingly many seem to react to that too. All this applies to chocolate drinks, mousses, sauces, anything cacao related and so on.

Cilantro: 4

- Histamine Intolerance Site: 😕 (yellow - medium histamine)

- Comments:

Cinnamon: 2

- Histamine Intolerance Site: 😕 (yellow - medium histamine)

- Comments: this is one of those ones where the major food list seem to disagree some say cinnamon is low histamine and some say it is high. From personal experience we have noted a reaction to histamine so we suggest acting very cautiously and we have given it a rating of 2 as reactions may vary from person to person.

Citrus Fruits: 1

- Histamine Intolerance Site: 😠 (red - high histamine)

- Comments: most citrus seems to be very high in histamine.

Clover: 2

- Histamine Intolerance Site: 😠 (red - high histamine)
- Comments:

Cloves: 5

- Histamine Intolerance Site: ☑ (green - low histamine)
- Comments: Low histamine.

Cocoa Butter And Cacao Butter: 2

- Histamine Intolerance Site: 😕 (yellow - medium histamine)
- Comments: Histamine-releasing. See our comments on 'Chocolate'.

Cocoa Drinks, Powder, Etc: 1

- Histamine Intolerance Site: 😠 (red - high histamine)
- Comments: See under 'Chocolate'.

Coconut And Coconut Derivatives: 4

- Histamine Intolerance Site: ☑ (green - low histamine)
- Comments: Some aspects of coconut can be high histamine, particularly coconut aminos. In addition, while most people seem to be okay with coconut there are a significant number of histamine intolerance people who do not get on well with it so test carefully. Coconut milks sometimes have a number of additives in them which

means that they go from being low histamine to high histamine say that it's something to look out for on the ingredients label.

Coffee: 3

- Histamine Intolerance Site: 😖 (yellow - medium histamine)

- Comments: Oh, this is something we could write a whole book about. Coffee massively divides people in the histamine intolerance community. About half of us seem to be able to tolerate it, and half of us don't. That does seem to be a benefit to seeking out low histamine, low mould, organic, low toxin coffees.

Coriander: 5

- Histamine Intolerance Site: ✅ (green - low histamine)
- Comments:

Corn Salad, Lamb's Lettuce: 5

- Histamine Intolerance Site: ✅ (green - low histamine)
- Comments:

Cornflakes: 5

- Histamine Intolerance Site: ✅ (green - low histamine)
- Comments: There are a number of foods that might be well-tolerated in terms of histamine intolerance but are going to be particularly good for your overall health. Let's

HISTAMINE INTOLERANCE FOOD LIST

put cornflakes into that category. We've given it a '5' as they should be low histamine as long as they don't have additives. But there are healthier breakfast options.

Courgette: 5

- Histamine Intolerance Site: ✓ (green - low histamine)
- Comments

Crab: 1

- Histamine Intolerance Site: 😠 (red - high histamine)
- Comments: see comments elsewhere on fish and seafood

Cranberry: 5

- Histamine Intolerance Site: ✓ (green - low histamine)
- Comments

Crawfish: 1

- Histamine Intolerance Site: 😠 (red - high histamine)
- Comments: Fish generally not tolerated well.

Crayfish: 1

- Histamine Intolerance Site: 😠 (red - high histamine)
- Comments: Fish generally not tolerated well.

Cream Cheeses: 3

- Histamine Intolerance Site: 😕 (yellow - medium histamine)

- Comments: see other comments on cheese. Organic is best.

Cream: 5

- Histamine Intolerance Site: ✅ (green - low histamine)

- Comments: Aim for grass-fed. If fermented, histamine levels rise.

Cress: 4

- Histamine Intolerance Site: 😕 (yellow - medium histamine)

- Comments

Cucumber: 5

- Histamine Intolerance Site: ✅ (green - low histamine)

- Comments: Note - this is fresh cucumber, not pickled. Anything pickled is a different story.

Cumin: 3

- Histamine Intolerance Site: 😡 (red - high histamine)

- Comments: The big lists seem to divert quite considerably around cumin. We love using it in our cooking and would hate to give it up and seem to react okay. However not everybody agrees that cumin is a suitable ingredient for those with histamine intolerance

Curry: 3

- Histamine Intolerance Site: 😕 (yellow - medium histamine)

- Comments: Clearly not all curries are created equal: Curry leaves are thought to be low histamine but curry powder high histamine. In addition you want to check for the level of spice and additives.

Dates: 3

- Histamine Intolerance Site: 😕 (yellow - medium histamine)

- Comments: Experts disagree on whether dates are high or low histamine. Test carefully. We've given them a '3' as we tolerate them generally speaking. Also note they are very high in sugar.

Dextrose: 5

- Histamine Intolerance Site: ✅ (green – low histamine)

- Comments

Dill: 4

- Histamine Intolerance Site: 😕 (yellow - medium histamine)

- Comments

Dragon Fruit: 5

- Histamine Intolerance Site: ✅ (green – low histamine)
- Comments

Dried Meat: 1

- Histamine Intolerance Site: 😠 (red - high histamine)
- Comments: Unfortunately, normally very high in histamine.

Dry-Cured Meats: 1

- Histamine Intolerance Site: 😠 (red - high histamine)
- Comments: Old and cured - that means high in histamine.

Duck: 5

- Histamine Intolerance Site: ✅ (green – low histamine)
- Comments

Egg White: 4

- Histamine Intolerance Site: 😕 (yellow - medium histamine)
- Comments: Cooked eggs without other ingredients can often be okay. Some believe that egg white can be mast cell activating. However The Histamine Intolerance Awareness Site notes; 'The theory, that egg white is a histamine releaser has been dismissed.' Many tolerate eggs and

especially egg yolks. Always buy organic and pasture-raised.

Egg Yolk: 3

- Histamine Intolerance Site: 😕 (yellow - medium histamine)
- Comments: See comments above. Always buy organic and pasture-raised.

Elderflower Cordial: 5

- Histamine Intolerance Site: ✅ (green – low histamine)
- Comments

Endive: 5

- Histamine Intolerance Site: ✅ (green - low histamine)
- Comments

Espresso: 3

- Histamine Intolerance Site: 😕 (yellow - medium histamine)
- Comments: We've given espresso its own slot in our food list, as it's better tolerated than regular coffee according to SIGHI. We're not so sure, but they know what they are talking about. Test carefully.

Fennel: 5

- Histamine Intolerance Site: ✅ (green - low histamine)

- Comments:

Fenugreek: 2

- Histamine Intolerance Site: 😠 (red - high histamine)

- Comments:

Feta Cheese: 3

- Histamine Intolerance Site: 😕 (yellow - medium histamine)

- Comments: For many, feta cheese falls into the soft cheese category and slightly better tolerated than many of the hard or blue veiny cheeses. Again this is a matter of considerable variance between different people. How confusing it is to have histamine intolerance when one person will react so badly to a particular Cheese and another person won't. We totally get this and that is why we ask you to test carefully.

Figs (Fresh Or Dried): 4

- Histamine Intolerance Site: 😕 (yellow - medium histamine)

- Comments: Fresh are likely to be lower histamine than dry.

Fish: 1

- Histamine Intolerance Site: 😠 (red - high histamine)

- Comments: All fish except freshly caught and frozen we list as high histamine. Fish also increases in histamine extraordinarily quickly. Certain fish, especially salmon, is okay if caught fresh, and then frozen quickly after catching. Fish freshly caught within an hour or frozen within an hour may well be better tolerated. Any fish in a fishmongers, or smoked gets a '1'.

Flaxseed (Linseed): 5

- Histamine Intolerance Site: ☑ (green – low histamine)
- Comments: Sprouted flaxseed is often even better tolerated than normal - but it costs more to buy.

Fructose (Fruit Sugar)

- Histamine Intolerance Site: ☑ (green - low histamine)
- Comments: It might be low histamine, but you want to avoid too much sugar.

Game (Meat): 4

- Histamine Intolerance Site: ☺ (yellow – medium histamine)
- Comments: Organic meat is best.

Garlic: 4

- Histamine Intolerance Site: ☺ (yellow – medium histamine)

- Comments: Garlic relatively well tolerated, although not 100% by everybody so it doesn't quite get a '5' rating.

Ginger: 4

- Histamine Intolerance Site: ✓ (green – low histamine)
- Comments

Goat's Milk: 5

- Histamine Intolerance Site: ✓ (green – low histamine)
- Comments

Goji Berry: 5

- Histamine Intolerance Site: ✓ (green – low histamine)
- Comments

Goose (Organic, Freshly Cooked): 5

- Histamine Intolerance Site: ✓ (green – low histamine)
- Comments

Gooseberry, Gooseberries: 5

- Histamine Intolerance Site: ✓ (green – low histamine)
- Comments:

Gouda Cheese: 1

- Histamine Intolerance Site: 🙁 (red – high histamine)

- Comments: See general comments under 'Cheese'.

Grapefruit: 1

- Histamine Intolerance Site: 😡 (red – high histamine)
- Comments: While many foods are on the allowed list with histamine intolerance this one is a disappointment - grapefruit normally seems to cause a reaction.

Grapes: 3

- Histamine Intolerance Site: ✅ (green – low histamine)
- Comments: Some lists don't agree the grapes are low histamine so we've given this a lower score. In addition they are very high in sugar.

Green Beans – See "Beans"

Green Peas: 3

- Histamine Intolerance Site: 😐 (yellow – medium histamine)
- Comments: peas are a weird one. We seem to tolerate them well, however having canvassed the histamine community many people do struggle with them. Mast Cell 360 lists green split peas and yellow split peas as low histamine, just "peas" as high histamine.

Green Tea: 3

- Histamine Intolerance Site: 😕 (yellow – medium histamine)

- Comments

Guava: 2

- Histamine Intolerance Site: 😡 (red – high histamine)

- Comments: High in oxalates.

Ham (Dried, Cured): 1

- Histamine Intolerance Site: 😡 (red – high histamine)

- Comments: Avoid processed meat, dried meat and cured meat. Will make your histamine intolerance worse.

Hazelnut: 3

- Histamine Intolerance Site: 😕 (yellow – medium histamine)

- Comments: Might be unlucky not to get a '4'. Test carefully but we consider one of the best nuts.

Hemp Seeds (Cannabis Sativa): 5

- Histamine Intolerance Site: ✅ (green – low histamine)

- Comments: We love hemp derivative and CBD products too.

Herbal Tea: 3

- Histamine Intolerance Site: 😕 (yellow – medium histamine)

- Comments: Depends on the tea and the individual ingredients. Please look up the individual ingredients in our list.

Honey: 5

- Histamine Intolerance Site: ✅ (green – low histamine)

- Comments:

Horseradish: 3

- Histamine Intolerance Site: 😕 (yellow – medium histamine)

- Comments

Juniper Berries (5)

- Histamine Intolerance Site: ✅ (green – low histamine)

- Comments

Kale: 5

- Histamine Intolerance Site: ✅ (green – low histamine)

- Comments: Kale listed as lower histamine on the major sites.

Kefir: 1

- Histamine Intolerance Site: 😣 (red – high histamine)
- Comments: High histamine as fermented. This could be lower histamine if you make it yourself with histamine-friendly bacteria.

Kelp: 1

- Histamine Intolerance Site: 😣 (red – high histamine)
- Comments

Kiwi: 3

- Histamine Intolerance Site: 😣 (red – high histamine)
- Comments: As you can see the Histamine Intolerance Site intolerance list kiwi as high histamine. However others disagree so we've given it a rating of three and would ask you to approach cautiously.

Kohlrabi: 4

- Histamine Intolerance Site: 😕 (yellow – medium histamine)
- Comments

Lamb: 5

- Histamine Intolerance Site: ✅ (green – low histamine)
- Comments: Must be organic and fresh. No leftovers.

Lamb's Lettuce, Corn Salad: 5

- Histamine Intolerance Site: ✅ (green – low histamine)
- Comments

Lard: 5

- Histamine Intolerance Site: ✅ (green – low histamine)
- Comments: fresh or frozen only.

Laurel, Bay Leaf: 3

- Histamine Intolerance Site: 🙁 (yellow – medium histamine)
- Comments:

Leek: 4

- Histamine Intolerance Site: 🙁 (yellow – medium histamine)
- Comments: likely to be low histamine

Lemon: See "Citrus Fruit"

Lentils: 2

- Histamine Intolerance Site: 😠 (red – high histamine)
- Comments. Some say lentils are actually low histamine, although high if tinned. We find them to be high histamine

Lettuce: 5

- Histamine Intolerance Site: ☑ (green – low histamine)
- Comments

Lime: 1

- Histamine Intolerance Site: 😠 (red – high histamine)
- Comments: More notes under 'Citrus'.

Lingonberry: 5

- Histamine Intolerance Site: ☑ (green – low histamine)
- Comments

Liquor – See Alcohol

Liquorice: 1

- Histamine Intolerance Site: 😠 (red – high histamine)
- Comments

Lobster: 1

- Histamine Intolerance Site: 😠 (red – high histamine)
- Comments: See notes under 'Fish'.

Loganberry: 2

- Histamine Intolerance Site: 😕 (yellow – medium histamine)

- Comments

Lychee: 5

- Histamine Intolerance Site: ✅ (green – low histamine)
- Comments: Must be fresh, not canned.

Macadamia: 4

- Histamine Intolerance Site: 😕 (yellow – medium histamine)
- Comments:

Malt extract: 1

- Histamine Intolerance Site: 😡 (red – high histamine)
- Comments

Malt: 1

- Histamine Intolerance Site: 😡 (red – high histamine)
- Comments: Includes barley malt and malt extract

Maltodextrin: 3

- Histamine Intolerance Site: ✅ (green – low histamine)
- Comments: Quite a considerable difference between major experts about whether maltodextrin is good for those who are histamine intolerant. Approach cautiously. While maltodextrin on its own may be lower histamine, the

end result may be higher histamine levels in the body. Check out 'sweeteners' for better natural alternatives.

Mandarin Orange: See "Citrus Fruit"

Mango: 4

- Histamine Intolerance Site: 😕 (yellow – medium histamine)

- Comments

Maple Syrup: 5

- Histamine Intolerance Site: ✅ (green – low histamine)

- Comments: Note previous comments about keeping sugar levels low for optimum health in relation to histamine intolerance.

Margarine: 1

- Histamine Intolerance Site: 😡 (red – high histamine)

- Comments: almost always contains sub-optimal ingredients.

Marrow: 5

- Histamine Intolerance Site: ✅ (green – low histamine)

- Comments

Mascarpone Cheese: 3

- Histamine Intolerance Site: 😕 (yellow – medium histamine)

- Comments: See other comments about soft cheeses. May be better tolerated than hard cheeses.

Mate tea: 1

- Histamine Intolerance Site: not listed

- Comments: The Histamine Intolerance Awareness Site lists mate tea under 'foods that have been reported to block the diamine oxidase (DAO) enzyme'

Melon: 4

- Histamine Intolerance Site: ✅

- Comments: The Histamine Intolerance Site lists melon as low histamine but please note, watermelon is listed in a different category as medium histamine and should be approached with caution

Milk: 5

- Histamine Intolerance Site: ✅ (green – low histamine)

- Comments: Includes, UHT, pasteurised. Milk powder and lactose-free milk may be higher in histamine.

Millet: 5

- Histamine Intolerance Site: ✅ (green – low histamine)

- Comments

Minced Meat: Fresh 5/Open Sale 3

- Histamine Intolerance Site: ☑ (green – low histamine)

- Comments: If eaten immediately after its production, then minced meat is a 5. However - and this is a big one - if it is then left then it can rise in histamine quicker than other forms of meat. There are some histamine-intolerant people who even buy their own mincer to avoid this issue. If you are not quite that committed yet (and we don't blame you if you aren't!) then look for the freshest mince with the longest best before date, and eat immediately or freeze. So we have given this one two scores, one for completely freshly ground, and one for open sale as it's hard to know the freshness and histamine levels of each individual portion.

Mint: 5

- Histamine Intolerance Site: ☑ (green – low histamine)
- Comments:

Morel: 2

- Histamine Intolerance Site: 😠 (red – high histamine)
- Comments

Morello Cherries: 4

- Histamine Intolerance Site: ☑ (green – low histamine)

- Comments: See other comments on 'Cherry' and 'Acerola'

Mozzarella Cheese: 4

- Histamine Intolerance Site: 😕 (yellow ~ medium histamine)
- Comments: See other comments on soft cheeses. Mozzarella is often well tolerated by many who are histamine intolerant but not everybody which is why we don't give it a top rating. Soft cheeses tend to be a better option than hard cheese or mouldy cheese.

Mulberry: 3

- Histamine Intolerance Site: 😕 (yellow ~ medium histamine)
- Comments

Mungbeans (Germinated, Sprouting): 2

- Histamine Intolerance Site: 😕 (yellow ~ medium histamine)
- Comments: See other comments on beans.

Mushrooms, Different Types: 2/3

- Histamine Intolerance Site: 😕 (yellow ~ medium histamine)
- Comments: another ingredient where opinion is divided. So much so that we give it a 2/3 rating. Please test carefully.

As you can see the Histamine Intolerance Site gives this a medium rating.

Mustard And Mustard Seeds: 2

- Histamine Intolerance Site: 😠 (red – high histamine)

- Comments

Napa Cabbage: 5

- Histamine Intolerance Site: ✅ (green – low histamine)

- Comments

Nectarine: 2

- Histamine Intolerance Site: 😕 (yellow – medium histamine)

- Comments: this is one where opinion varies. On SIGHI it is ranked as low histamine. On the respected site SFGATE it is noted as high histamine. And the Histamine Intolerance Site sensibly comes down in the middle. We give it a 2 rating, and ask you to test carefully.

Nettle Tea: 2

- Histamine Intolerance Site: not listed

- Comments: Alison Vickery quotes excellent studies which suggest nettle is a potent antihistamine (working at the H1 receptor) and mast cell stabilizer. So this may be a good option. However, approach cautiously as some still react to nettle tea.

Nori Seaweed: 1

- Histamine Intolerance Site: 😠 (red – high histamine)
- Comments: Poorly tolerated, expect symptoms.

Nutmeg: 2

- Histamine Intolerance Site: 😕 (yellow – medium histamine)
- Comments: Nutmeg flower and nutmeg flower oil seem to be tolerated more effectively.

Nuts: 1-5 (See Individual Nuts For More Details)

- Histamine Intolerance Site: 😕 (yellow – medium histamine on average although individual nuts listed separately)
- Comments: Nuts hugely depend, both from nut to nut, and on each individual batch in terms of freshness. One of the things we consistently find with nuts is that the lower our histamine levels are generally, the more we can tolerate them. Conversely, if we are in the middle of a flareup, we avoid nuts as bitter experience has shown that it causes more of a reaction. So please check each individual nut to see if it is listed for more detail.

Oats: 5

- Histamine Intolerance Site: ✅ (green – low histamine)
- Comments: Oats are a real staple for those with histamine intolerance. But what about other oat products. Oat milk can be a good option when out and about and ordering

coffee for example. But always be mindful of other ingredients in oat drinks. For instance a number of oat milks have lots of additives whereas others only have three or four ingredients. So pick a good one - organic if possible.

Olive Oil: 5

- Histamine Intolerance Site: ✅ (green – low histamine)

- Comments: We believe a better choice when extra virgin. Organic extra virgin olive oil (or Organic EVOO as we like to call it) is even better.

Olives: 2

- Histamine Intolerance Site: 😕 (yellow – medium histamine)

- Comments: As good as olive oil is, frustratingly olives come up much lower in our list.

Onion: 4

- Histamine Intolerance Site: 😕 (yellow – medium histamine)

- Comments:

Orange: 1

- Histamine Intolerance Site: 😡 (red - high histamine)

- Comments: most citrus seems to be very high in histamine.

Oregano: 5

- Histamine Intolerance Site: ☑ (green – low histamine)
- Comments: Both fresh and dried seems to be tolerated well.

Ostrich: 5

- Histamine Intolerance Site: ☑ (green – low histamine)
- Comments: Note other comments about fresh meat elsewhere. No leftovers.

Oyster: 1

- Histamine Intolerance Site: ☹ (red – high histamine)
- Comments

Pak Choi: 5

- Histamine Intolerance Site: ☑ (green – low histamine)
- Comments

Palm Kernel Oil: 5

- Histamine Intolerance Site: ☑ (green – low histamine)
- Comments

Palm Oil: 5

- Histamine Intolerance Site: ☑ (green – low histamine)

- Comments: Always go for a sustainable brand - not for health but the environment.

Papaya: 1

- Histamine Intolerance Site: 😠 (red – high histamine)
- Comments: One of the fruits most likely to cause a reaction.

Paprika, Hot: 1

- Histamine Intolerance Site: 😠 (red – high histamine)
- Comments: Not to be confused with sweet paprika

Paprika, Sweet: 5

- Histamine Intolerance Site: ✓ (green – low histamine)
- Comments: Not to be confused with hot paprika

Parsley: 5

- Histamine Intolerance Site: ✓ (green – low histamine)
- Comments

Parsnip: 5

- Histamine Intolerance Site: ✓ (green – low histamine)
- Comments: We love the humble parsnip. Be warned, it can go off quite quickly though, so eat fresh.

Passion Fruit: 5

- Histamine Intolerance Site: no info
- Comments

Peach: 5

- Histamine Intolerance Site: ☑ (green – low histamine)
- Comments: We like to buy, chop and freeze and use in small portions in desserts.

Peanuts: 1

- Histamine Intolerance Site: 😡 (red – high histamine)
- Comments: One of the worst nuts for histamine

Pear: 3

- Histamine Intolerance Site: 😕 (yellow – medium histamine)
- Comments: If canned then likely to be higher in histamine than fresh.

Peas (Green): 3

- Histamine Intolerance Site: 😕 (yellow – medium histamine)
- Comments: peas are a weird one. We do well with them, however having canvassed the histamine community many people do struggle with them. Mast Cell 360 lists

---

green split peas and yellow split peas as low histamine, just "peas" as high histamine.

Pea Shoots (Or Pea Sprouts): 5

- Histamine Intolerance Site: ✓ (green - low histamine)
- Comments: Believed to be histamine-lowering. A superb addition to your shopping list.

Pepper: 2

- Histamine Intolerance Site: 😠 (red – high histamine)
- Comments: Comes up as high histamine in many lists, but some people seem to tolerate. This applies to white and black pepper.

Peppermint Tea: 5

- Histamine Intolerance Site: ✓ (green - low histamine)
- Comments

Pickled Food: 1

- Histamine Intolerance Site: all 😠 (red – high histamine)
- Comments: All pickled food gets a 1 in our list. Watch out for pickled gherkins in burgers!

Pine Nuts: 3

- Histamine Intolerance Site: 😕 (yellow – medium histamine)

- Comments

Pineapple: 1

- Histamine Intolerance Site: 😠 (red – high histamine)
- Comments: On the Healing Histamine Site, author Yasmina got to the point where she could eat high histamine foods whenever she wanted, though she **always** chose high nutrient, healing foods, and didn't eat them at every meal. She notes how important it is to reintroduce 'healthy' higher histamine foods such as pineapple once you start to feel better, and we whole-heartedly agree.

Pistachio: 4

- Histamine Intolerance Site: 😕 (yellow – medium histamine)
- Comments

Plum: 2

- Histamine Intolerance Site: 😕 (yellow – medium histamine)
- Comments

Pomegranate: 5

- Histamine Intolerance Site: ✅ (green – low histamine)
- Comments: Thought by many to be histamine lowering so an excellent option for you. Pomegranate seeds are delicious in salads.

Poppy Seeds: 4

- Histamine Intolerance Site: 😕 (yellow – medium histamine)

- Comments

Porcino Mushroom: 1

- Histamine Intolerance Site: 😟 (red – high histamine)

- Comments

Pork: 5

- Histamine Intolerance Site: ✅ (green – low histamine)

- Comments: As long as organic and freshly cooked - pork gets a 5. Non-organic would get a lower score. No leftovers.

Potato: 5

- Histamine Intolerance Site: ✅ (green – low histamine)

- Comments: above applies to all potato types. Includes sweet potato too.

Poultry Meat: 5

- Histamine Intolerance Site: ✅ (green – low histamine)

- Comments: As long as organic and very fresh- poultry gets a 5. Non-organic would get a lower score. No leftovers.

Prawn: 1

- Histamine Intolerance Site: 😠 (red – high histamine)
- Comments:

Processed Cheese: 1

- Histamine Intolerance Site: 😠 (red – high histamine)
- Comments: the words *processed* and *cheese*, both = high histamine

Prune: 4

- Histamine Intolerance Site: 😕 (yellow – medium histamine)
- Comments

Psyllium Seed Husks: 5

- Histamine Intolerance Site: ✅ (green – low histamine)
- Comments:

Pulses: 1

- Histamine Intolerance Site: 😠 (red – high histamine)
- Comments: See "beans" for more info

Pumpkin Seed Oil: 5

- Histamine Intolerance Site: ✅ (green – low histamine)
- Comments:

Pumpkin Seeds: 4

- Histamine Intolerance Site: ✅ (green – low histamine)
- Comments: Very occasionally we notice a reaction to pumpkin seeds. Most of the recognised sources say they are low histamine. Also applies to pumpkin seed oil.

Pumpkin: 4

- Histamine Intolerance Site: ✅ (green – low histamine)
- Comments: The respected site Fact vs Fitness puts pumpkin on their restricted list.

Quail: 5

- Histamine Intolerance Site: ✅ (green – low histamine)
- Comments: Organic, freshly cooked if possible.

Quail Eggs: 5

- Histamine Intolerance Site: ✅ (green – low histamine)
- Comments: A good egg option.

Quinine: 2

- Histamine Intolerance Site: 😕 (yellow – medium histamine)
- Comments:

Quinoa: 5

- Histamine Intolerance Site: ☑ (green – low histamine)
- Comments: A good gluten-free option.

Rabbit: 5

- Histamine Intolerance Site: ☑ (green – low histamine)
- Comments: Organic, freshly cooked meat is typically safe.

Raclette Cheese: 1

- Histamine Intolerance Site: 😠 (red – high histamine)
- Comments:

Radish: 5

- Histamine Intolerance Site: ☑ (green – low histamine)
- Comments: Applies to red and white radishes.

Raisins (If No Sulphur): 5

- Histamine Intolerance Site: ☑ (green – low histamine)
- Comments: As long as no sulphur you should find these are okay. However most raisins have added sunflower oil.

Rapeseed Oil (Called Canola Oil In US): 2

- Histamine Intolerance Site: ☑ (green – low histamine)

- Comments: We've marked this down as we've noticed at times it can cause inflammation. But you might well find it agrees with you.

Raspberry: 2

- Histamine Intolerance Site: 😠 (red – high histamine)
- Comments:

Raw Milk: 5

- Histamine Intolerance Site: ✓ (green – low histamine)
- Comments:

Red Cabbage: 5

- Histamine Intolerance Site: ✓ (green – low histamine)
- Comments: See more under 'Cabbage'.

Red Wine Vinegar: 1

- Histamine Intolerance Site: 😠 (red – high histamine)
- Comments: All vinegar listed as high histamine apart from Apple Cider Vinegar. See other vinegars for more details.

Redcurrants: 5

- Histamine Intolerance Site: ✓ (green – low histamine)
- Comments:

Rhubarb: 4

- Histamine Intolerance Site: 😕 (yellow – medium histamine)
- Comments:

Rice: 5

- Histamine Intolerance Site: ✅ (green – low histamine)
- Comments: Please note that whilst freshly cooked rice is what we are referring to here, pre-cooked packaged rice may have different histamine levels.

Rice Cakes: 5

- Histamine Intolerance Site: ✅ (green – low histamine)
- Comments:

Rice Milk: 4

- Histamine Intolerance Site: 😕 (yellow – medium histamine)
- Comments: Watch out for added ingredients in rice milks. As a rule of thumb the few ingredients for the better.

Rice Noodles: 5

- Histamine Intolerance Site: ✅ (green – low histamine)
- Comments:

Ricotta Cheese: 4

- Histamine Intolerance Site: 😕 (yellow – medium histamine)

- Comments: Tends to be one of the best tolerated of the cheeses. As this is a soft cheese it may be a better option for you.

Rooibos Tea: 5

- Histamine Intolerance Site: ✓ (green – low histamine)

- Comments:

Roquefort Cheese: 2

- Histamine Intolerance Site: 😕 (yellow – medium histamine)

- Comments:

Rosemary: 5

- Histamine Intolerance Site: ✓ (green – low histamine)

- Comments:

Rum: 1

- Histamine Intolerance Site: 😠 (red – high histamine)

- Comments: Alcohol is high histamine, and please check other notes on alcohol in this book. We do find that some alcohols are slightly less inflammatory than others. Rum suits some better, but is high histamine all the same.

Rye: 3

- Histamine Intolerance Site: 😕 (yellow – medium histamine)
- Comments:

Sage: 5

- Histamine Intolerance Site: ✅ (green – low histamine)
- Comments: Includes sage tea.

Salami: 1

- Histamine Intolerance Site: 😣 (red – high histamine)
- Comments: Cured meats should be avoided, and unfortunately salami comes into this category. Cured meats are more generally considered poor for health as well as high histamine.

Salmon: 1 (Although Read Comments)

- Histamine Intolerance Site: 😣 (red – high histamine)
- Comments: Salmon deserves some special comments here because while all fish tends to score very low on histamine levels, salmon is one that if it is caught and frozen quickly tends to be tolerated much more effectively. We have found some good salmon brands which deliver frozen. Wild-caught and organic are best.

Sauerkraut – See "Pickled Food"

Sausages Of All Kinds: 1

- Histamine Intolerance Site: 😠 (red – high histamine)
- Comments:

Savoy Cabbage: 4

- Histamine Intolerance Site: 😕 (yellow – medium histamine)
- Comments:

Schnapps: 1

- Histamine Intolerance Site: 😠 (red – high histamine)
- Comments: See 'Alcohol'.

Seafood: 1

- Histamine Intolerance Site: 😠 (red – high histamine)
- Comments: All seafood except freshly caught and frozen we list as high histamine. Fish also increases in histamine extraordinarily quickly. Certain fish can be okay if caught fresh, and then frozen quickly after catching. Fish freshly caught within an hour or frozen within an hour may well be better tolerated. Any fish in a fishmongers, or smoked scores a '1'.

Seaweed: 1

- Histamine Intolerance Site: 😡 (red – high histamine)
- Comments:

Sesame: 4

- Histamine Intolerance Site: 😕 (yellow – medium histamine)
- Comments: Sesame seeds also seem to be tolerated.

Sheep's Milk, Sheep Milk: 5

- Histamine Intolerance Site: ✅ (green – low histamine)
- Comments:

Shellfish: 1

- Histamine Intolerance Site: 😡 (red – high histamine)
- Comments: See comments on fish and seafood.

Shrimp: 1

- Histamine Intolerance Site: 😡 (red – high histamine)
- Comments:

Smoked Fish: 1

- Histamine Intolerance Site: 😡 (red – high histamine)
- Comments: Fish score low on our scale. Smoked fish - even lower.

Smoked Meat: 1

- Histamine Intolerance Site: 😠 (red – high histamine)
- Comments:

Snow Peas – See "Green Peas"

Soft Cheese: 3

- Histamine Intolerance Site: 😕 (yellow – medium histamine)
- Comments: See comments under 'Cheese'.

Sour Cherry: 4

- Histamine Intolerance Site: ✅ (green – low histamine)
- Comments: See other comments on 'Cherry'

Sour Cream: 3

- Histamine Intolerance Site: 😕 (yellow – medium histamine)
- Comments:

Soy (Soy Beans, Soy Flour): 1

- Histamine Intolerance Site: 😠 (red – high histamine)
- Comments: Includes soy milk, soya milk, and other soy drinks

Soy Sauce: 1

- Histamine Intolerance Site: 😠 (red – high histamine)
- Comments:

Sparkling Wine: 1

- Histamine Intolerance Site: 😠 (red – high histamine)
- Comments: More in the 'Alcohol' section.

Spelt: 5

- Histamine Intolerance Site: ☑ (green – low histamine)
- Comments: Check for gluten if avoiding gluten.

Spinach: 1

- Histamine Intolerance Site: 😠 (red – high histamine)
- Comments: One of those foods that is generally considered 'healthy' but unfortunately high in histamine.
- listed, Nopales cactus listed as low histamine
- Comments:

Spirits: 1

- Histamine Intolerance Site: 😠 (red – high histamine)
- Comments: See comments on 'Alcohol'.

Squashes: 5

- Histamine Intolerance Site: ☑ (green – low histamine)
- Comments:

Stevia: 5

- Histamine Intolerance Site: ☑ (green – low histamine)
- Comments: Our favourite natural sweetener. Includes stevia leaves, liquid, powder.

Stinging Nettle: 1

- Histamine Intolerance Site: 😠 (red – high histamine)
- Comments: Alison Vickery quotes some excellent studies which suggest nettle is a potent antihistamine (working at the H1 receptor) and mast cell stabilizer. Approach cautiously as some still react to nettle tea.

Strawberry: 1

- Histamine Intolerance Site: 😠 (red – high histamine)
- Comments: Mast Cell 360 notes that strawberries may be tolerated in in very small amounts (ie 1 strawberry)

Sugar: 5

- Histamine Intolerance Site: ☑ (green – low histamine)
- Comments: Sugar may be low histamine but is not good for those with health issues. When it comes to sugar, try

natural alternatives. Stevia, and monk fruit are the best natural alternatives. Inulin is another one to try.

Sunflower Oil: 2

- Histamine Intolerance Site: 😕 (yellow – medium histamine)

- Comments: We've marked this down as we've noticed at times it can cause inflammation. This also goes for Rapeseed/Canola oil But you might well find it agrees with you and some sites note it is generally low histamine.

Sunflower Seeds: 2

- Histamine Intolerance Site: 😣 (red – high histamine)

- Comments: We also notice sunflower seeds cause a general inflammation related to histamine, but this is anecdotal and you may well have a different experience.

Sweetcorn: 5

- Histamine Intolerance Site: ✅ (green – low histamine)

- Comments:

Sweet Potato: 5

- Histamine Intolerance Site: ✅ (green – low histamine)

- Comments: above applies to other potatoes

Sweeteners (If Natural): 5

- Histamine Intolerance Site: ☑ (green – low histamine)

- Comments: Stevia, and monk fruit are the best natural alternatives. Stevia really is delicious. Warning - you need a very small quantity for a sweet taste. Inulin is another natural sweetener to try. Artificial sweeteners are not a '5' but a '1' and have their own category.

Tap Water: 5

- Histamine Intolerance Site: ☑ (green – low histamine)

- Comments: Filtered water is preferable.

Tea, Black: 1

- Histamine Intolerance Site: 😠 (red – high histamine)

- Comments: The Histamine Intolerance Awareness Site lists black tea under 'foods that have been reported to block the diamine oxidase (DAO) enzyme'

Thyme: 5

- Histamine Intolerance Site: ☑ (green – low histamine)

- Comments: Includes common thyme, German thyme, garden thyme

Tiger nut: 5

- Histamine Intolerance Site: ☑ (green – low histamine)

- Comments: Not actually a nut - this is an excellent option for a nut replacement. It is quite sweet but higher in carbs and sugar than most nuts.

Tomato: 1

- Histamine Intolerance Site: 😠 (red – high histamine)
- Comments: Includes tomato juice. On the Healing Histamine Site, author Yasmina notes how important it is to reintroduce 'healthy' higher histamine foods such as tomato once you start to feel better.

Trout: 1

- Histamine Intolerance Site: 😕 (yellow – medium histamine)
- Comments: Worth a comment as SIGHI notes freshwater brown trout, brook trout, and rainbow trout are low histamine. That's not our experience but may be for others.

Tuna: 1

- Histamine Intolerance Site: 😠 (red – high histamine)
- Comments: all canned food is high in histamines. Tuna also tends to be high in heavy metals.

Turkey: 5

- Histamine Intolerance Site: ✅ (green – low histamine)
- Comments: See other comments about preferably eating organic and freshly cooked. No leftovers.

Turmeric: 5

- Histamine Intolerance Site: ☑ (green – low histamine)
- Comments: Inflammation-fighting and low histamine.

Turnip: 4

- Histamine Intolerance Site: 😕 (yellow – medium histamine)
- Comments: Includes turnip greens, turnip roots and turnip cabbage.

Vanilla: 3

- Histamine Intolerance Site: 😕 (yellow – medium histamine)
- Comments: Includes vanilla, vanilla extract, vanilla pod, vanilla powder, vanilla sugar. Please note - vanilla essence is often in alcohol, which means that it would score considerably lower.

Venison: 4

- Histamine Intolerance Site: ☑ (green – low histamine)
- Comments:

Vinegar: Apple Cider Vinegar: 3

- Histamine Intolerance Site: 😕 (yellow – medium histamine)

- Comments: Apple vinegar is the lowest of all vinegars in histamine. Also look for verjus if you cannot tolerate ACV.

Vinegar: Balsamic: 1

- Histamine Intolerance Site: 😠 (red – high histamine)
- Comments:

Vinegar: Distilled White Vinegar: 1

- Histamine Intolerance Site: 😠 (red – high histamine)
- Comments:

Walnut: 1

- Histamine Intolerance Site: 😠 (red – high histamine)
- Comments: One of the most problematic of nuts when it comes to histamine. Also applies to walnut oil.

Watercress: 5

- Histamine Intolerance Site: ✅ (green – low histamine)
- Comments: Potentially histamine-lowering. Alison Vickery notes a study which showed that the peppery-flavoured watercress inhibits 60% of all histamine released from mast cells.

Watermelon: 1

- Histamine Intolerance Site: 😕 (yellow – medium histamine)

- Comments: The Histamine Intolerance Site lists melon as low histamine but please note, watermelon is listed in a different category as medium histamine and should be approached with real caution. Many people do not agree with watermelon when considering histamine. Fact vs Fitness puts watermelon on their 'allowed' list, so it's something you may want to approach with caution.

Wheat: 3

- Histamine Intolerance Site: 😕 (yellow – medium histamine)
- Comments: Wheat in itself gets a medium writing in our book. However many people observe giving up gluten does help their overall histamine and wellness levels so this is something you may want to consider

Wheat Germ: 1

- Histamine Intolerance Site: 😡 (red – high histamine)
- Comments:

Whey: 4

- Histamine Intolerance Site: ✅ (green – low histamine)
- Comments:

White Button Mushroom: 2

- Histamine Intolerance Site: 😕 (yellow – medium histamine)

- Comments: See 'Mushrooms' for more on mushrooms.

White Onion: 4

- Histamine Intolerance Site: 😕 (yellow – medium histamine)
- Comments:

White Vinegar, Spirit Vinegar: 1

- Histamine Intolerance Site: 😡 (red – high histamine)
- Comments: Approach vinegars with caution.

White Wine Vinegar: 1

- Histamine Intolerance Site: 😡 (red – high histamine)
- Comments:

Wild Rice: 5

- Histamine Intolerance Site: ✅ (green – low histamine)
- Comments: See more comments on 'Rice'.

Wine: 1

- Histamine Intolerance Site: 😡 (red – high histamine)
- Comments: Comments: Alcohols are some of the most problematic things you can consume on a low histamine diet. Wines are often extremely difficult although some low-histamine wines can be found. But note the DAO-blocking element in the 'Alcohol' section. Alcohols contain

histamine-degrading enzymes, but some rums, tequilas and Tito's Vodka may be purer than others. We have seen some claims online that plain vodka, gin and white rum are all low in histamine - these may be better options than other alcohols, but they still may block your DAO enzyme and therefore cause a histamine reaction.

Yam: 5

- Histamine Intolerance Site: ☑ (green – low histamine)
- Comments:

Yeast: 2

- Histamine Intolerance Site: 🙁 (yellow – medium histamine)
- Comments: Varies from batch to batch. Applies to fresh and dried, approach with extreme caution.

Yeast Extract: 1

- Histamine Intolerance Site: 😠 (red – high histamine)
- Comments: The Histamine Intolerance Awareness Site notes yeast extract is a DAO inhibitor and is therefore not suitable on a low-histamine diet.

Yogurt/Yoghurt: 1

- Histamine Intolerance Site: 😠 (red – high histamine)

- Comments: Unfortunately, almost always high histamine. You could try making your own batch with low histamine bacteria.

Zucchini: 5

- Histamine Intolerance Site: ✅ (green – low histamine)
- Comments: Also known as courgette.

Made in the USA
Middletown, DE
08 November 2021